CHAIR YOGA

FOR WEIGHT LOSS

28-Day Challenge to Shed Belly Fat, Regain Mobility and Flexibility with Low-Impact Seated Exercises in just 10 Minutes a Day

By

Semine T.

Table of Contents

Introduction

The World Obesity Atlas has revealed alarming statistics: 38% of the global population is currently grappling with obesity and overweight issues. We gain weight when there is an imbalance between how much we consume and how much our body uses. However, is it possible to balance these impacts? What if exercise does not mean daily gym sessions for hours but a few seated exercises? What if we adopt an effective way to control this imbalance - not by high-impact workouts in the gym, but by low-impact seated positions?

This book offers that solution: Chair Yoga.

The gym can be intimidating for many people, with its vast array of machines and numerous members going about their workouts. For years, I knew I needed to exercise more, but I was uncomfortable with lifting weights or running. I eventually found an alternative - chair yoga. It's a low-impact workout that is customizable and easy on your body. This makes it perfect for anyone looking to improve their quality of life without feeling any added pressure or risk of injury.

Recent studies have shown that chair yoga can improve flexibility and strength as much as regular yoga. This book aims to help you lay a foundation for using your muscles, which may have been dormant for a long time. The exercises have been designed to ensure no potential risk of overloading or falling. Once you find balance in the chair, you can gradually incorporate ankle weights, hand weights, or resistance bands into your routine.

This book asks you to spare 10-minutes of your day for 28 days. You will be proud of yourself for developing a habit of standing in front of the mirror, seeing an energized body and a shining smile, and saying, "I did it." It is just the first step, and it takes time. For that, the easy-to-follow structure of this book will guide you.

In this book, you will find:

- **Beginner, intermediate, and advanced level routines:** Chair yoga is suitable for any age group; as adults, no matter your age or fitness level, we have poses that fulfill any criteria.
- **Exercises with step-by-step instructions:** Whether you want to lose weight, shed belly fat, or enhance mobility and flexibility, our targeted 10-minute daily routine exercises cover it all.
- **A holistic approach:** We care for your physical and mental well-being by providing nutrition, mindful eating, and stress management guidance with a complete 28-day chart.

Before we take our chairs and start yoga, let's be clear on what chair yoga stands for.

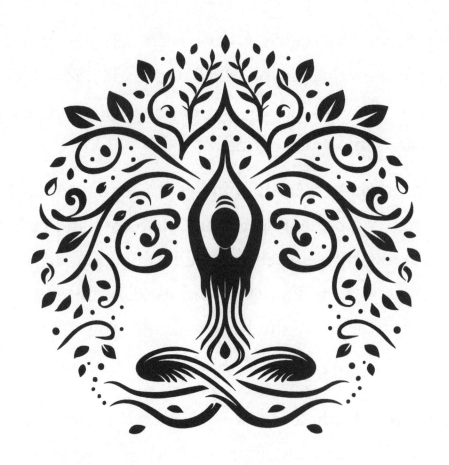

CHAPTER 1

INTRODUCING CHAIR YOGA

Your body asks for a yoga break from your desk, couch, and car. Imagine experiencing all of the benefits of yoga, including relaxation and the ability to lose few pounds while remaining comfortably seated. This chapter will walk you through chair yoga, the benefits of this exercise, and how you can succeed in 28 days.

What is Chair Yoga?

Chair yoga means performing yoga with the help of a chair, thus making it accessible for everyone. It is also a gentle form of yoga because most poses are seated. Whether you do yoga with a chair or on a mat, the exercises focus on mindful breathing, attention to your thoughts, and being present. While doing this yoga, you have a supportive partner, i.e., your sturdy chair, which provides a safe way to do exercises for people of all age levels. Even if you have never done yoga, chair yoga is an excellent start to mindful movements.

Benefits of Chair Yoga

In modern life, we are glued to our chairs, beds, couches, and cars. We all crave a way to reverse the stiffness, aches, and stress of this sedentary lifestyle. What if I do it while sitting in a chair? Why should I choose chair yoga? What can these mindful poses give me that those fancy poses cannot?

To answer these questions, let's consider its benefits:

- Research has shown that participants noticed that their shoulders, necks, and lower backs became flexible and less stiff after adopting chair yoga exercises.
- Much research is being done to study the body-mind connection, which suggests that chair yoga reduces stress and anxiety levels.
- Other research published in the International Journal of Yoga supports the idea that chair yoga builds a strong core and increases balance in older adults.

- Not everyone can jump right into a downward-facing dog pose. Still, a 2018 review published in the Journal of Disability and Rehabilitation showed chair yoga was beneficial for people with physical limitations or injuries as it let them enjoy the benefits of yoga without any pressure.
- Similarly, a research paper published in Frontiers in Psychology has stated that chair yoga affects our mood, as the study participants felt more energetic and had an optimistic view of life after adopting to chair yoga interventions.

Chair Yoga for Weight Loss

Traditional weight loss methods may seem daunting. You may feel sore and discouraged after high-impact workouts or do not like going to crowded gyms. Chair yoga is an alternative that gives you the same result with low-impact seated positions. A study conducted in 2021 has shown that combining chair yoga with a healthy diet leads to significant weight loss, particularly in belly fat.

These are the ways how it does so:

- Studies have suggested that all kinds of yoga impact our metabolism positively. Metabolism is the rate at which our body burns calories. When it is improved, our body burns calories even at rest.
- As mentioned, chair yoga exercises target our major muscle groups, improving our metabolic system.
- Chair yoga improves the flexibility of body, which means you can add a greater range of motion to daily activities. The more we

move our body, the more calories we burn.

- Chair yoga works alongside mindful eating, which means choosing healthier food and managing portions of our meals.
- Chronic stress causes weight gain. When we follow a daily chair yoga routine, we also focus on deep breathing and meditation, which manage our stress hormones.

Low-impact seated exercises with chairs are a safe choice for everyone, regardless of age or fitness level. You might take it as your starting point to build mobility and flexibility, opt for weight loss, and recover from injuries.

Success in 28 Days

Choosing a 28-day time frame is not random. Research has shown that it takes 21 days to develop a new habit, with an extra week for reinforcement. After 28 days, you will see noticeable change in your mobility, strength, flexibility, and endurance. Here are some ways to ensure your success with 10-minutes per day for 28 days (rest days will be included too):

- Instead of saying, "I want to lose weight," target a specific area like your belly fat.
- Set a millstone, such as feeling strength in your shoulder and hip muscles.
- Be specific about your goal. For example, you should improve your balance.
- Be specific about daily sessions or reps and modifications of poses.

- Record yourself while doing exercises to gain confidence.
- Find a partner to make it more fun.

The key is to remain consistent. Now that you have gained enough knowledge, we will see what you need to start. Before that, let's learn some practical strategies to maximize your yoga's results.

Strategies for Getting Maximum Results

Follow these strategies to get the maximum results from your chair yoga for losing weight.

- **Practice it daily:** It's essential to make it a daily must-do. Substitute longer and less frequent workouts with shorter sessions, saving yourself time and effort.
- **Inhale deeply and burn calories:** In chair yoga, mindful breathing should be part of every pose, making exercise more efficient and mindful.
- **Consider your core your powerhouse:** It stabilizes your poses and helps maintain balance while burning many calories, as it is almost continuously engaged.
- **Look for progressions:** As you master your chair yoga skills, think of more challenging poses to try. Listen to your body's signals. Determine whether you are ready for new challenges or need to stop.
- **Proper nutrition:** While chair yoga may not feel like an exhausting workout, it still burns calories when combined with proper nutrition.

- **Beyond chair yoga:** While chair yoga will become a significant part of your daily or weekly routine, always vary your workouts.

- **Practice at your own pace:** Practice with people who understand you, witness your growth, and support you. We all have our own pace; find yours.

- **Make it simple:** The significant advantage of chair yoga is the simplicity with which one may do modifications. The beauty of yoga lies in the freedom with which it can be adjusted. If holding a straight posture for an extended period is difficult, some variations include using a pillow behind your back or utilizing a supportive chair where you can lean back.

- **Use online resources:** Listen to your body and avoid stretching to the extent you feel pain. In addition to this book, online resources can also provide videos showing exactly how chair yoga should be done.

- **Consult your doctor:** You can always make changes according to your preferences. However, always check with your doctor before you exercise, especially if you have a pre-existing medical condition.

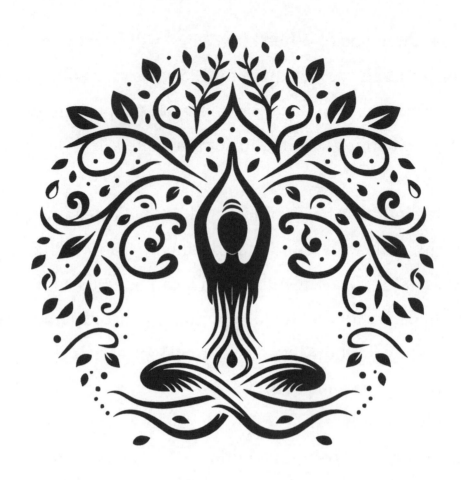

CHAPTER 2

BEFORE YOU START

This chapter sets the stage and guides you through the proper use of a chair, the essentials of chair yoga, and the starting and ending rituals, which include warm-up, cool-down, and breathing exercises.

Finding Your Chair

Find a chair with a sturdy base and a flat, firm seat to sit in the ideal position, keeping your knees at a 90-degree angle.

Consider these:

- If you need extra support for balancing poses or getting up and down, choose a chair with an armrest.
- Choose a straight-backed chair for twists and spinal stretches if you have back issues.
- Choose a comfortable chair that allows you to move freely and gain balance.

Chair Yoga Essentials

Chair yoga is done with minimal equipment. However, you can use props to get comfortable and modify certain poses. These basic yoga essentials may include:

- **Yoga Blocks:** Yoga blocks are available in multiple sizes. They may help elevate your hands or enhance your stretch levels, allowing you to do so securely and comfortably.
- **Yoga Straps:** At times, chair poses require reaching one's feet or hand to the foot. If that is a flexibility obstacle, you can use a yoga strap! Straps make up for the lost additional stretch by ensuring proper alignment without straining. In this way, you can focus on the core benefits of the pose.

- **Blanket:** Use a warm, comfortable blanket for extra padding.

It is up to you to use whatever you need to make the exercise as effective as you can.

Starting and Ending Rituals

Nothing is better than creating starting and ending rituals for any physical exercise. It gives structure to your exercise routine. Here is how you can do it while doing chair yoga.

Starting Rituals (Warm-up)

- Before you start, find a calm place, using some candles, essential oils, or music as per your taste.
- Calm your mind and ask yourself your intention behind doing yoga.
- Take four deep breaths and relax your body.
- Warm-up is a must. It is essential to avoid any injury and prepare your body for motion. This book has many poses for all levels, from beginner to advanced. The beginner-level poses will warm your body and target your neck, spine, shoulders, arms, hips, and legs.

Closing Ritual (Cool-down)

- A closing ritual takes your body back to a resting state. The transition must be in the form of exercises to avoid any adverse effects afterward. You can use seated forward folds, pigeon poses, or spinal twists given in the book.

- Use the deep breathing technique and relax.
- You can also lie down on your back and be present.
- Reflect on your experience of each yoga day and write it down in a journal.

Deep Breathing

Adopt this deep breathing technique before starting yoga, during each exercise, and while cooling down.

- Sit straight in the chair and put your hands on your stomach.
- Keep your feet flat on the surface.
- Keep your eyes closed, breathe through the nose, feel hands moving away from the body, and breathe out through the mouth.

We know about chair yoga, we have the chair and chair yoga essentials, we have understood the starting and closing rituals, and we have learned to do deep breathing. It is time to sit in the chair and start.

Get the Most out of Your Chair Yoga Practice

Keep in mind the following key information to get the best results out of your chair yoga exercises.

- The chair should be durable enough to allow you to sit with your knees at a 90-degree angle.

- If you need extra support for balancing or getting up and down, you can use a chair with armrests for balance.

- Look for a straight-backed chair for back stretches and twists to help you with back pain.

- Props are not necessary but can help with comfort and modification. Always use props whenever you need extra support and cannot reach a pose without it.

- Yoga straps are perfect for modifying poses and increasing flexibility.

- A warm up takes the workout to the next step and helps prevent injury.

- Include the cool-down exercises in your routine. Although you may feel stiff or sore, the cool-down helps your body relax and avoid any injury.

- Breathe in through your nose and breathe out with your mouth wide open, comfortably and quietly.

- Warm-up and cool-down exercises should last about 3 -4 minutes. A brief warm-up or cool-down and a few breaths are enough.

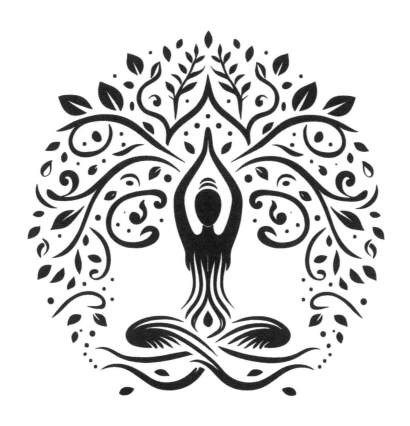

CHAPTER 3

CHAIR YOGA FOR BELLY FAT

We will start with our first goal, which is fat loss and reducing belly fat. This chapter introduces you to chair yoga poses and exercises that will engage all your body muscles and target belly fat. These include beginner-level warm-up poses, intermediate-level core strength poses, and advanced-level cardio workout poses on a chair while focusing on mindful breathing. Take your time and step up the first ladder; we have much to do with our chair.

Beginner Level

At this level, we will do gentle and simple movements and stretches to prepare our core for the upcoming poses.

Cat-Cow Stretch

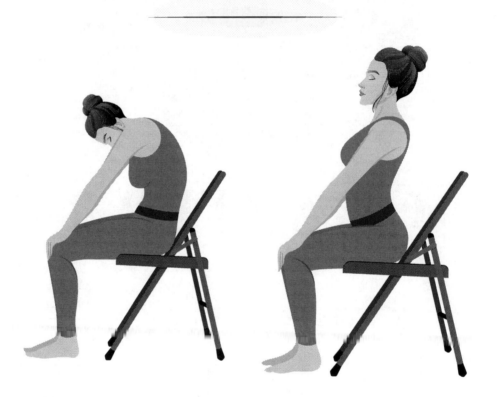

Instructions

1. Get your sturdy chair and sit comfortably.
2. Place your hands on your thighs or knees while keeping your feet firm.
3. Breathe in and arch your back while opening your chest outward and lifting your chin.
4. Exhale and curl your back inward while pointing your chin toward your chest.

5. Repeat it 2-3 times.

Benefits

- Warm-up
- Improves flexibility
- Relieves stress
- Treats back pain
- Burns calories

Modification: To feel more comfortable, use a short chair or place a blanket under your feet or behind your back.

Safety Tip: Avoid excessive arching or curling of your back.

Seated Side Stretch

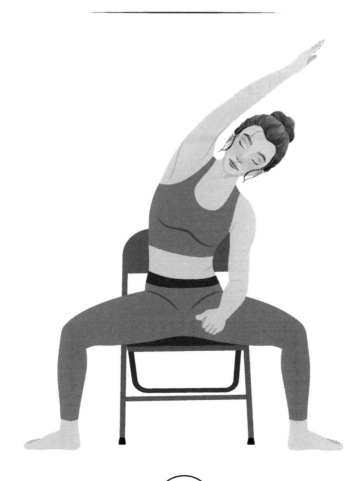

Instructions

1. Get yourself comfortable in the chair.

2. Place your hands on your knees while your feet are firmly planted on the floor.

3. Stretch your legs and move them away from each other.

4. Raise your right hand high above your head. You can support yourself with your left hand on your leg or the arm of the chair.

5. Breathe in as you raise your arm as high as you can, then release as you slowly bend to the left as far as you can. If you can, raise your gaze to your hand.

6. Take three breaths and hold. Continue on the opposite side.

Benefits

- Flexible muscles
- Strong shoulders, hips, and back
- Better posture
- Warm-up

Modification: You can hold a yoga strap looped around your foot for support.

Safety Measure: Keep your back stretched throughout the pose.

Forward Bend

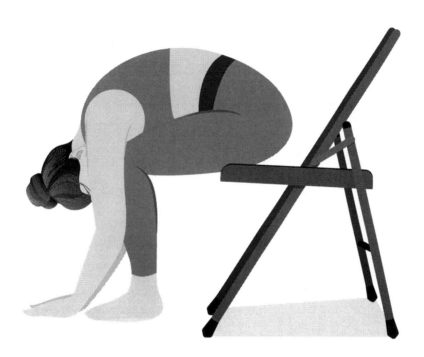

Instructions

1. Sit on a sturdy chair and make sure your spine is straight.
2. Keep your feet flat and firm on the ground, and lean forward to touch the ground.
3. Fold your torso between your stretched legs.
4. Round your slightly curved spine and drop the head to face the ground.
5. Slowly move back to the original seated position.
6. Repeat it 3-4 times.

Benefits

- Improves hamstring and spine flexibility
- Strengthens core muscles
- Increases blood flow
- Burns calories
- Helps in stress and tension reduction

Modification: You can modify this pose by doing a forward bend and slowly and gently interlacing your fingers behind your back to open your chest.

Safety Tip: Ensure your chair does not tip over as you bend forward.

Seated Spinal Twists

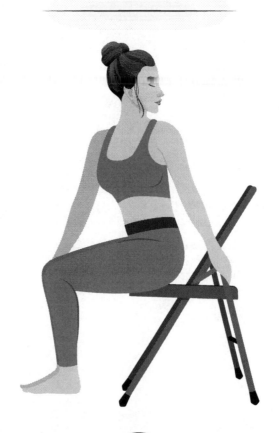

Instructions

1. Sit in the chair with your back straight and feet firm on the ground.
2. Keep your legs at a 90-degree angle.
3. Twist your upper body toward the left side and hold onto the back of your chair with the left hand.
4. Hold this position and take 2-3 deep breaths.
5. Move your body back to the center and relax.
6. Move and do the same twist to your right side in the same manner.

Benefits

- Warm-up
- Improves range of motion
- Spinal flexibility and mobility

Modification: After twisting your upper body to one side, you can hold the chair with both hands.

Safety Tip: Ensure that your lower body does not twist and keep supporting your lower back.

Intermediate Level

At this level, we will focus on more dynamic movements.

Seated Leg Lifts

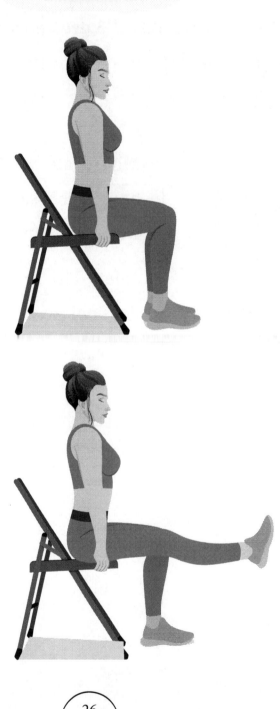

Instructions

1. Sit in the chair and keep your back straight and feet firm on the ground.
2. Keep your legs at a 90-degree angle.
3. Lift one of your legs and hold it straight, then hold it in this position for 2-3 deep breaths.
4. Focus on your breaths while you inhale or exhale.
5. Lower your leg and repeat this for the other leg.

Benefits

- Increases balance
- Strengthens core
- Strenghthens hips and legs
- Targets larger muscles to help burn more calories

Modification: When you find balance and feel confident, lift both legs and take 2-3 breaths while holding them up in the air.

Safety Tip: Ensure that your legs and back are straight.

Chair Eagle Pose

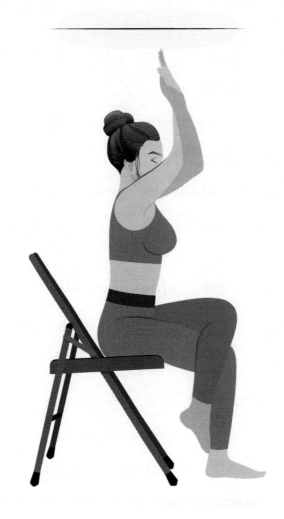

Instructions

1. Feel comfortable in the chair and relax.
2. Lift your elbows while keeping your shoulders straight and away from your ears.
3. Cross your left leg over your right thigh while bringing your thighs closer and squeezing together.
4. Hook the fingers of your left foot behind the right foot ankle.
5. Release your breath and place your right arm beneath your left, bending your elbows and pointing your fingers upward.

6. Bring the back side of both hands toward each other and press them against each other.

7. Slightly lift the elbows.

8. Hold for 2-3 breaths.

9. Uncross your legs and arms to come back to the original position.

10. Repeat this position starting with the opposite hand and leg.

Benefits

- Lower body strength
- Upper body strength
- Hip mobility
- Engages muscles

Modification: You can modify this pose by lifting one leg straight in front of you and keeping the other at a 90-degree angle.

Safety Tip: Please avoid this pose if you have any elbow, hip, or ankle injury.

Seated Cow Face

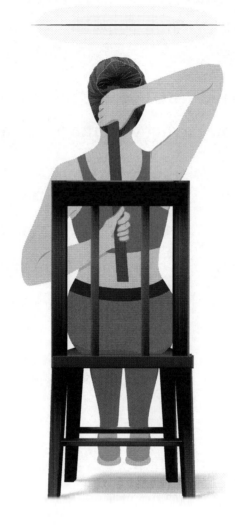

Instructions

1. Sit in the chair and keep your back straight and feet firm on the ground.
2. Keep your legs at a 90-degree angle.
3. Hold one corner of the strap in your right hand and lift it straight, pointing upward.
4. Bend your right elbow, and bring your right hand, holding the strap toward your back.

5. Now, you can hold the other side of the strap with your left hand to bring it to your midline.

6. Hold this position and breathe evenly for 2-3 breaths.

7. Release both hands and relax.

8. Repeat the steps starting with the left hand.

Benefits

- Improves posture
- Improves flexibility
- Stretches almost every part of the body
- Reduces belly fat

Modification: You can do this pose without a prop or strap.

Safety Tip: Do some warm-up exercises before doing this pose.

Advanced Level

We have reached a challenging and more exciting level where we will add more resistance and intense exercises.

Chair Boat Pose

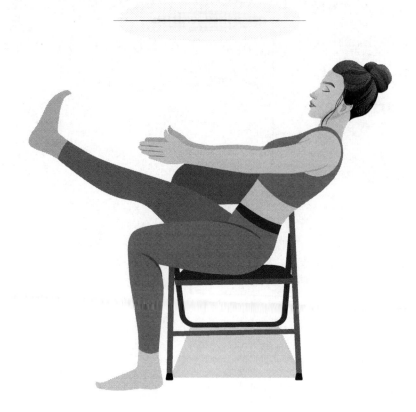

Instructions

1. Sit comfortably on the chair and relax.
2. Ensure that your back does not touch the back of the chair.
3. Slowly lift your right leg with the fingers of the right foot pointing to the ceiling and bring your leg to the level of your chest.

4. Keep the other arm at a 90-degree angle and your foot firm on the ground.

5. Lift your arms and stretch them straight, pointing in the same direction as your right leg.

6. Hold this position for 2-3 deep breaths.

7. Slowly bring down your hands and right leg and relax briefly.

8. Repeat it with the left leg.

Benefits

- Strengthens core
- Improves balance and focus
- Increases range of motion
- Highly effective in burning belly and hip fat

Modification: You can lift both legs to take this pose to the next level.

Safety Tip: Ensure that you do not curl your spine.

Chair Plank

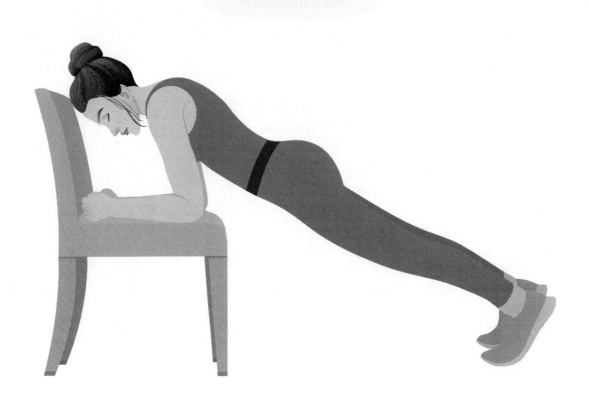

Instructions

This pose is different and unique. We will do plank but with a chair.

1. Find a sturdy chair and ensure it does not move.

2. Put your elbows on the chair and stretch the lower body.

3. Keep your spine straight; it will engage your core.

4. Keep your legs and back straight and stretched to form a straight line from head to heels.

5. Hold this position, inhale, and exhale for 2-3 deep breaths.

6. To return to the original position, slowly move your knees toward your elbows and reach a standing position.

Benefits

- Highly effective in weight loss
- Engages core muscles
- Increases balance and coordination
- Improves metabolism

Modification: You can place your hands on the chair instead of elbows.

Safety Tip: Ensure that you maintain a straight line with your body. If you find it challenging, give yourself some time and do it again.

Chair Reverse Warrior

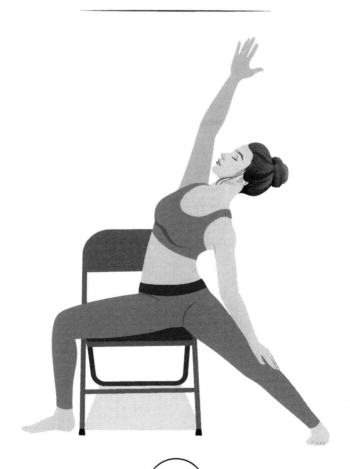

Instructions

1. Relax and recover from previous poses by sitting comfortably.
2. Keep your posture straight and move toward the left end of the chair.
3. Now, take your right leg out toward the right side of the chair and keep it at a 90-degree angle.
4. Move the left leg toward the left side of the chair and lengthen it to stretch it straight.
5. Lift your right arm toward the ceiling and place your left hand on the left knee.
6. Now, inhale and exhale slowly and move your right arm over your head toward the left side of the body.
7. Bend your upper body alongside the movement of the right arm to stretch your belly muscles.
8. Take 2-3 deep breaths.
9. Slowly take your right arm down and repeat the pose, starting with the left arm and left leg.

Benefits

- Stretches muscles
- Burns belly fat
- Improves flexibility
- Strengthens core

Modification: You can move your hand over your head more to take it to another level.

Safety Tip: Ensure you balance yourself well on the chair before starting this pose.

Seated Bicycle Crunches

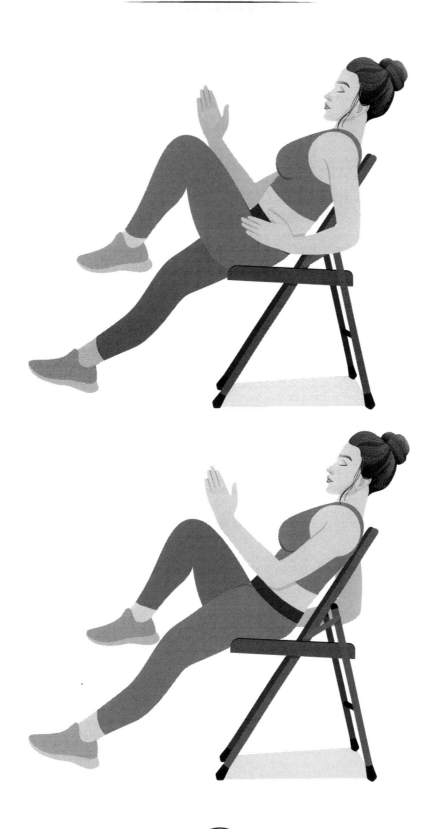

Instructions

1. Feel comfortable on the chair and relax.

2. Be mindful of your environment as we are moving toward an advanced level.

3. Lift both arms and stretch them in front of you.

4. Keep them straight and move your left leg toward your body by bending your knee.

5. Lift your right arm and bend it at a 45-degree angle with your body.

6. Now lower the left leg and right arm; get your right leg ready to move toward your body and your left arm bending at a 45-degree angle.

7. Gradually increase the speed of your legs and hand movement and take alternative turns.

8. Do this 10-15 times, and remember to take deep breaths.

9. Slowly decrease the speed to go back to the original position.

Benefits

- Increases mobility
- Provides cardio workout
- Burns fat
- Increases muscle flexibility
- Improves metabolism

Modification: To increase variation and endurance, you can leave the stretched leg in the air, a few inches above the ground.

Safety Tip: Do not suddenly increase the speed and intensity of your movements.

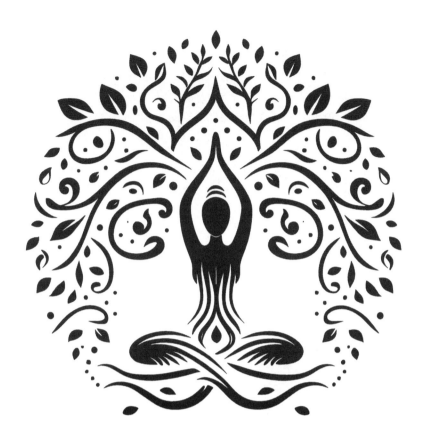

CHAPTER 4

CHAIR YOGA
FOR MOBILITY

Due to the wide range of options available, Chair Yoga is well-suited to anyone, regardless of their fitness level or level of expertise. This chapter will be divided into three sections: beginner, intermediate, and advanced. Each division will include step-by-step guidance for multiple sitting poses to increase your mobility.

Beginner Level

Use these exercises to warm yourself up.

Seated Neck Stretch

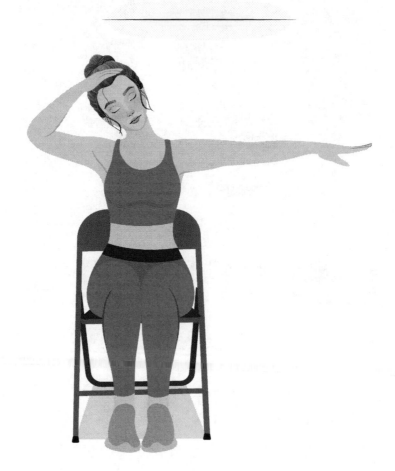

Instructions

1. Ensure that you are comfortable while sitting in the chair.
2. Keep your thighs close to each other and your legs at a 90-degree angle.
3. Slowly lift both arms and bring them parallel to the ground.
4. Bend your right arm and hold your head with the right hand.

5. Slowly and gently move your head with your hand toward the right side.

6. Hold this position for 2-3 breaths.

7. Slowly release your head and repeat this position with the left hand.

Benefits

- Improves neck mobility
- Reduces neck tension

Modification: You can keep the other hand down and point toward the ground.

Safety Tip: Ensure your posture is straight and the neck stretch is gentle.

Seated Shoulder Rolls

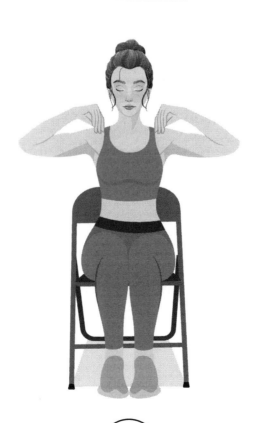

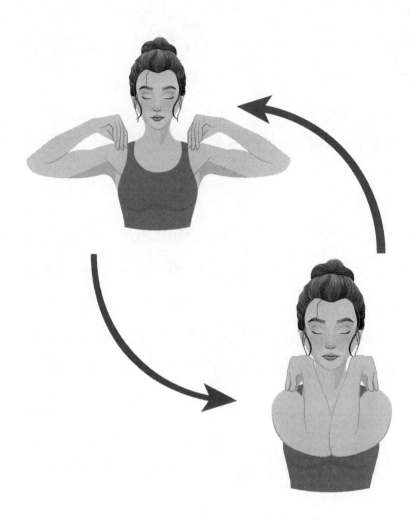

Instructions

1. Sit with a straight posture and relax.
2. Keep your legs at a 90-degree angle.
3. Now lift your arms and put your right-hand fingers on the right shoulder and your left-hand fingers on the left shoulder.
4. Now, rotate your elbows forward.
5. Form complete circles so that your elbows touch each other.
6. Remember to keep breathing and focusing on your breaths.
7. Make 5-10 circles.

Benefits

- Improves shoulder mobility
- Reduces shoulder tension
- Warms up the shoulder joints

Modification: You can rotate circles forward and backward.

Safety Tip: Ensure that your back is not curved.

Forward Bend Hamstring Stretch

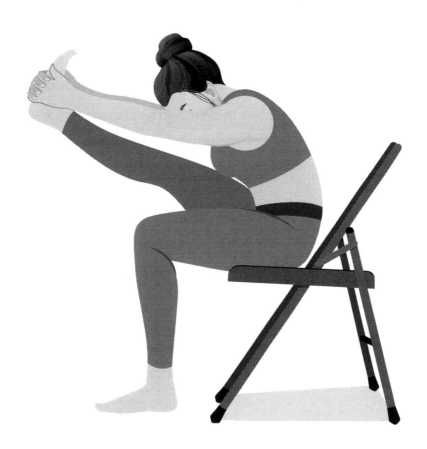

Instructions

1. Sit with a straight posture and relax your shoulders.

2. Keep your legs at a 90-degree angle.

3. Slowly raise your right leg and keep it straight and stretched.

4. Hold your right foot with both hands.

5. Keep your head down to stretch your neck.

6. Take 2-3 breaths. Inhale and exhale, and focus on your breaths.

7. Slowly raise your head, leave your foot, and bring your leg to the original position.

Benefits

- Improves hamstring flexibility
- Lengthens the back muscles
- Reduces lower back pain

Modification: You can lift both legs simultaneously to take it to an advanced level.

Safety Measure: Ensure that there is no bend in the knee.

Seated Hip Circles

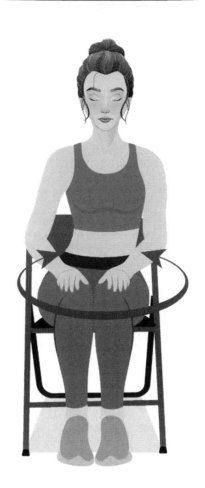

Instructions

1. Sit comfortably and keep your upper body in a vertical position.
2. Keep your legs at a 90-degree angle. You can bring them close to each other or keep them at shoulder length.
3. Slowly rotate three complete circles with your hips clockwise.
4. Keep breathing.
5. Now reverse the rotation and complete three circles anti-clockwise.
6. Slowly move back to the original position.

Benefits

- Improves hip mobility
- Makes the hip joints flexible
- Reduces hip pain

Modification: Gradually increase the size of circles to improve the range of motion.

Safety Tip: Ensure your back is not curved and your shoulders do not bend.

Intermediate Level

Now that you are comfortable with beginner-level poses take one step further.

Seated Neck Rolls

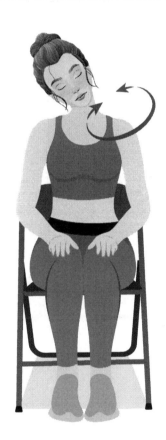

Instructions

1. Sit comfortably in the chair and place your hand on the thighs with your legs at a 90-degree angle.
2. Drop your head toward the right and feel a stretch in the neck.
3. Inhale and release your breath by rotating your head forward until it reaches the left side.

4. Inhale and rotate your head until it reaches the right side again.

5. Keep rotating for 4-5 breaths.

6. Repeat this by starting from the left side of your body.

Benefits

- Improves neck mobolity in multiple directions
- Reduces neck tension

Modification: Lift both arms and bring them in parallel positions to the ground while rotating your neck.

Safety Tip: Ensure that the rotation is smooth and slow initially.

Chair March

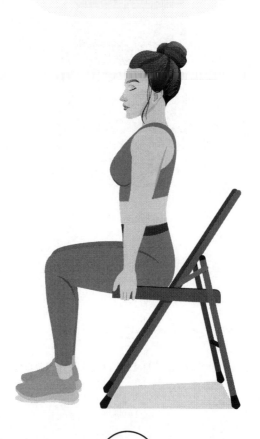

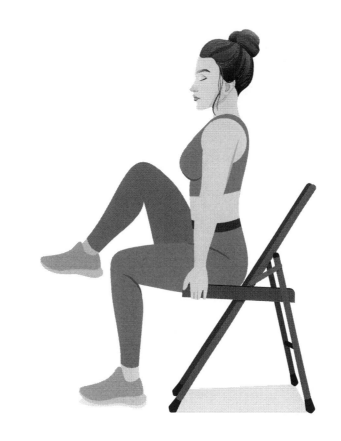

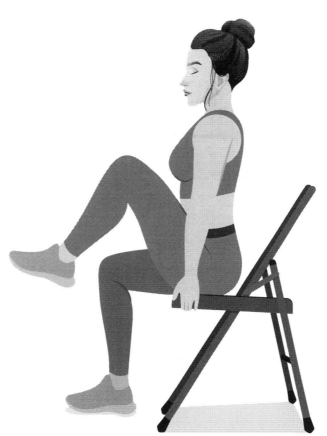

Instructions

1. Sit in a comfortable position and keep your back straight.

2. Keep your arm straight on both sides.

3. Inhale and slowly lift your right leg in a bending position.

4. Keep your stomach engaged and tight.

5. Exhale and drop the right leg while raising your left leg.

6. Keep taking turns until it looks like a march.

7. Do 10-15 marches while taking deep breaths.

Benefits

- Improves circulation
- Increases heart rate
- Warms up the legs
- Provides low-impact exercise

Modification: You can hold weights in your hands to build endurance.

Safety Measure: Do not arch or curl your back.

Chair Squats

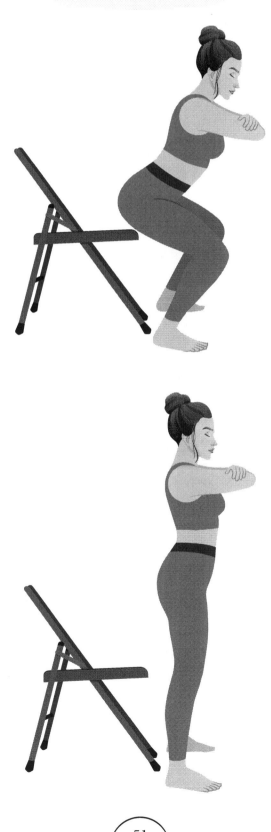

Instructions

1. Sit straight in the chair and keep your feet apart at shoulder's length.
2. Touch your right hand with your left shoulder and your left hand with your right shoulder.
3. Keep your elbows forward and straight.
4. Leave your sitting position, bend your knees, and move upward.
5. Create an arch in the back and inhale while standing up.
6. Now, come to the sitting position while exhaling.
7. Do this to 4-5 times.

Benefits

- Strengthens legs
- Improves balance
- Increases range of motion in the knees

Modification: You can hold weights to make it more advanced.

Safety Measure: Avoid this if you have knee pain.

Cross Body Punch

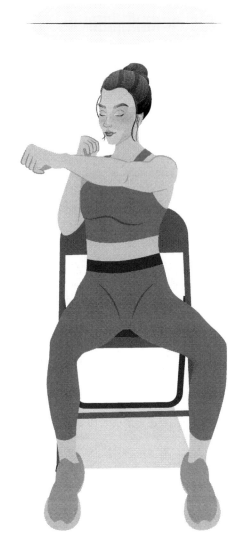

Instructions

1. Sit in the chair with your legs apart and back straight.

2. Do not bend your shoulder; keep your feet firm on the ground.

3. Bend your right arm so your right fist is close to your chin.

4. Inhale and lift your left arm by stretching forward and making a fist with your hand while moving it to the right side of the body.

5. Exhale while bending your left arm so your left hand comes close to your chin.

6. Now, inhale and stretch your right arm.

7. Keep doing these movements for 10-15 times.

Benefits

- Improves coordination
- Strengthens upper body
- Increases range of motion in the shoulders

Modification: Hold light weights to increase resistance.

Safety Measure: Ensure that your movements are controlled and rhythmic.

Advanced Level

Be bold and try some poses that test your yoga enthusiasm.

Reach out to Your Thigh

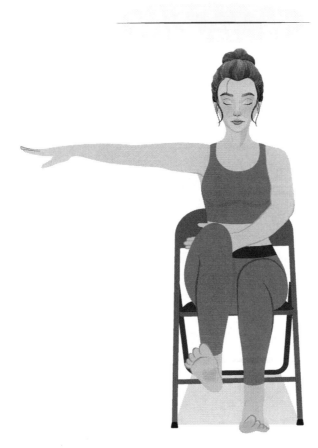

Instructions

1. Sit straight in the chair and keep your legs at a 90-degree angle and away from each other.
2. Lift your right hand and move it to the right side of the chair to bring it in a parallel position to the ground.
3. Now, put your left hand on the right thigh.
4. Slowly lift your right leg from the ground.

5. Hold this position for 2-3 deep breaths.

6. Repeat this yoga pose with the opposite leg and arm.

Benefits

- Improves balance
- Incrases flexibility in the side waist and legs
- Stretches the core

Modification: You can lift both your arms and legs simultaneously.

Safety Tip: Ensure that your belly and back are tight.

Chair Mountain Pose

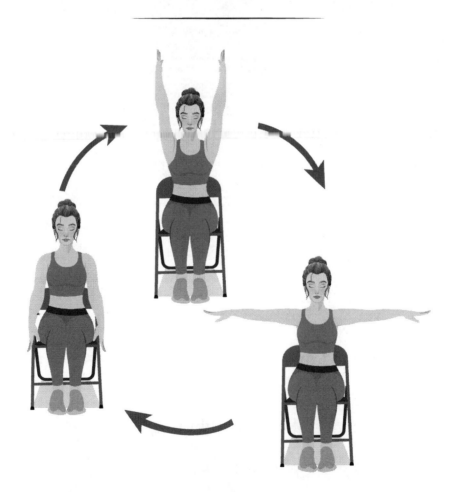

Instructions

1. Sit comfortably in the chair and bring your legs closer to each other.
2. Stretch both arms along the sides of your chair and feel like reaching the ground.
3. Slowly lift both arms, pointing them toward the ceiling.
4. Keep your upper body stretched and inhale.
5. Now, bring your arm parallel to the ground while exhaling.
6. From there, bring your arms down to the side.
7. Repeat this pose for 4-5 breaths.

Benefits

- Improves posture
- Strengthens core
- Increases flexibility in the spine

Modification: You can lift both legs while lifting your arms to make it more advanced.

Safety Measure: Ensure no arch or curl is in the upper body.

Chair Bicep Dips

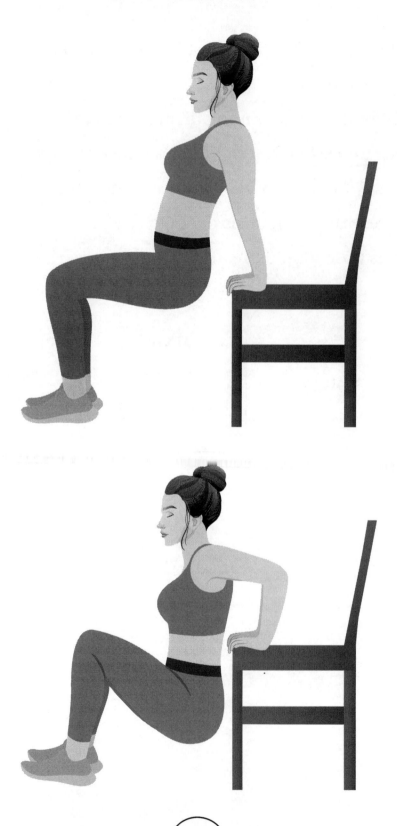

Instructions

1. Find a stable and sturdy chair as we will take its support to do biceps dips.

2. Roll your shoulders back and open up your chest.

3. Bring your hands underneath your shoulders on the chair.

4. Inhale while taking your legs out and keeping your knees bent.

5. Now exhale while bending the elbows and lowering your body down.

6. Now, inhale and move your body up by stretching your arms.

7. Repeat this movement for 3-4 breaths.

Benefits

- Strengthens biceps
- Improves upper body strength

Modification: You can lengthen and stretch your legs instead of bending from your knees.

Safety Measure: Ensure you do not shrink your shoulders while going down.

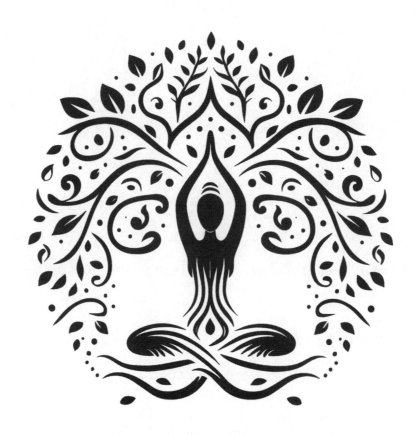

CHAPTER 5

CHAIR YOGA
FOR FLEXIBILITY

In this chapter, you will find various exercises to increase your body's flexibility. We will start with light warm-ups to bring your muscles into good working order. Afterward, we will move to the advanced poses to target your hamstrings, back, and shoulders, all while seated. Once you've done working through this chapter, you will improve your range of motion, muscle relaxation, and proper posture.

Beginner Level

Use these exercises to warm yourself up.

Seated Hamstring Stretch

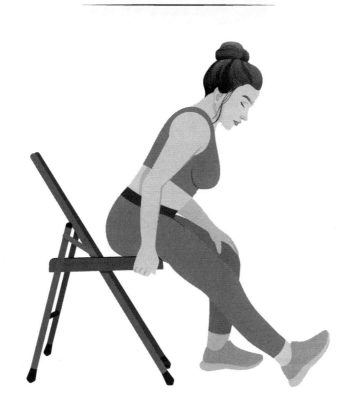

Instructions

1. Sit in a relaxing position in the chair.
2. Move toward the front edge of the chair and hold the chair with your right hand.
3. Keep the left leg at a 90-degree angle while stretching the right leg.
4. Touch the heel of your foot to the ground.
5. Lean forward and keep your spine straight.
6. Hold this position for 3-4 breaths.

7. Move back the stretched leg and repeat this with the opposite leg.

Benefits

- Improves flexibility in the hamstrings
- Reduces risk of injury
- Improves posture
- Improves blood circulation
- Reduces muscle soreness

Modification: Lean forward while stretching your back and holding your foot with your hand.

Safety Tip: Ensure that you do not bend your knee.

Seated Hero's Pose

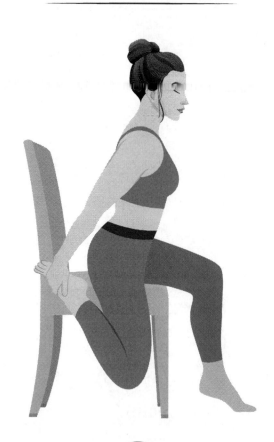

Instructions

1. Ensure that you use a stable chair.

2. Move to the right edge of the chair and keep your left leg at a 90-degree angle.

3. Raise your right heel and touch the ground with your fingers.

4. Now bend your right leg backward and hold your right foot in the right hand.

5. Stretch your chest outward and breathe slowly.

6. Hold this position for 3-4 breaths.

7. Bring the bent leg forward and repeat this with the opposite leg.

Benefits

- Stretches the calves and ankles
- Improves hip and ankles flexibility
- Strengthens core muscles
- Improves balance

Modification: You can use a yoga strap or towel around the arch of your foot.

Safety Measure: Ensure your chair does not fall toward the right side.

Seiated Inner Thigh Stretch

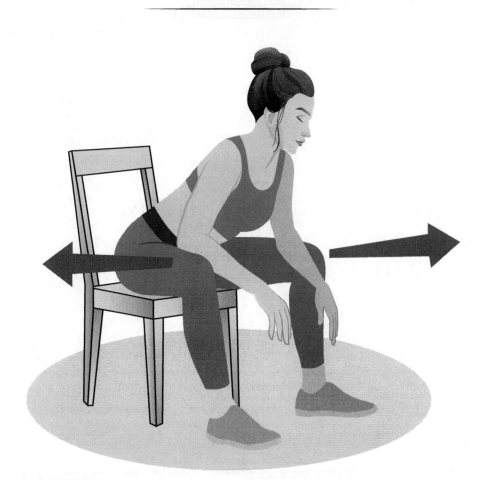

Instructions

1. Sit relaxed with both legs at a 90-degree angle.

2. Now, move your legs away from each other and stretch them.

3. Keep the feet firm on the ground.

4. Lean forward and keep your back stretched and straight.

5. Put your elbows near the knees and push the legs in the opposite direction.

6. Hold this position for 3-4 breaths.

7. Now, gently move your legs close to each other.

Benefits

- Stretches the inner thigh muscles
- Improves hip mobility
- Improves posture

Modification: You can convert this pose into a butterfly stretch by placing your feet on the table.

Safety Tip: Do not push your limits while stretching your legs.

Intermediate Level

Now that you are comfortable with beginner-level poses take one step further.

Seated Ankle Circles

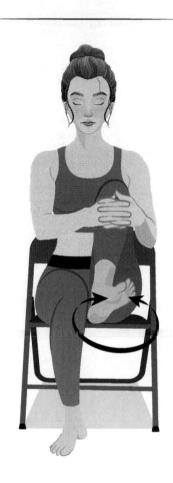

Instructions

1. Start this pose by sitting in a relaxed position.
2. Keep your back straight and your feet at a 90-degree angle.
3. Slowly bend your left leg so your knee touches your chest.
4. Use both hands to raise your leg and hold it with both hands.
5. Rotate your left foot and make small circles.

6. Keep breathing and complete 5-8 circles.

7. Take your leg down and repeat this exercise for the other leg.

Benefits

- Improves ankle mobility
- Increases circulation in the legs
- Relieves pain and stiffness in the ankles

Modifications: You can raise both legs simultaneously.

Safety Tips: If you have any knee injury, avoid this pose.

Seated Shoulder Twists

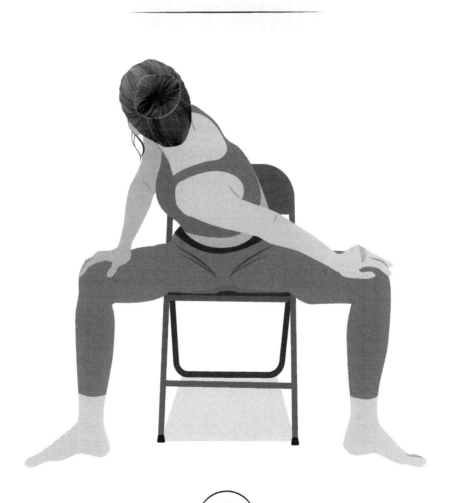

Instructions

1. Sit in the chair with your back stretched and place your hands on your knees.

2. Now, slowly move your legs to the sides of the chair so that your thighs become parallel to the ground.

3. Place your hands on your knees and lean forward.

4. Now move your upper body toward the right so that your shoulders come a 90-degree to the ground.

5. Stretch your legs further while pushing with your hands.

6. Hold this position for 4-5 breaths and repeat by moving to the other side.

Benefits

- Improves shoulder and spine mobility
- Reduces pain in the upper body and shoulders
- Improves posture

Modification: You can raise your hand and move toward your shoulder twist.

Safety Measure: Ensure that your back is stretched throughout this position.

Goddess Pose

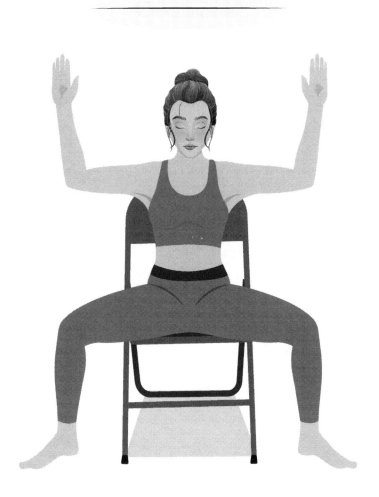

Instructions

1. Sit in the chair with your back stretched and place your hands on your knees.
2. Now, slowly move your legs to the sides of the chair so that your thighs become parallel to the ground.
3. Raise your heel and touch the ground with your fingers.
4. Raise your arms and hold them parallel to the ground, then bend them as your fingers point upward to the ceiling.
5. Do not bend your shoulders and move out your chest.

6. Hold this position for 3-4 deep breaths and slowly come to the original relaxing pose.

Benefits

- Strengthens inner thighs and outer hips
- Improves hip mobility
- Improves balance and stability

Modification: You can keep moving your arms forward and backward in the way that your forearms touch each other.

Safety Tip: Do not arch or curl the back.

Advanced Level

Be bold and try some poses to push yourself.

Chair Warrior II Pose

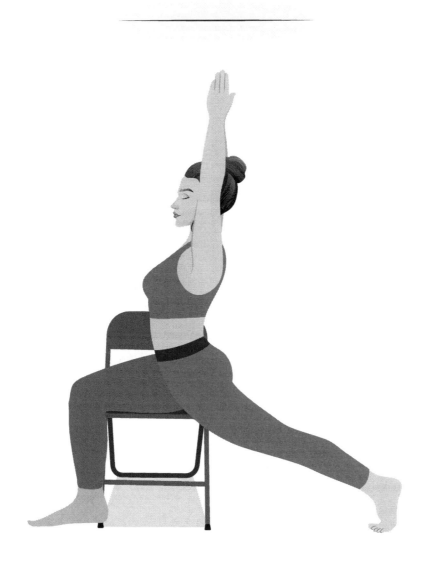

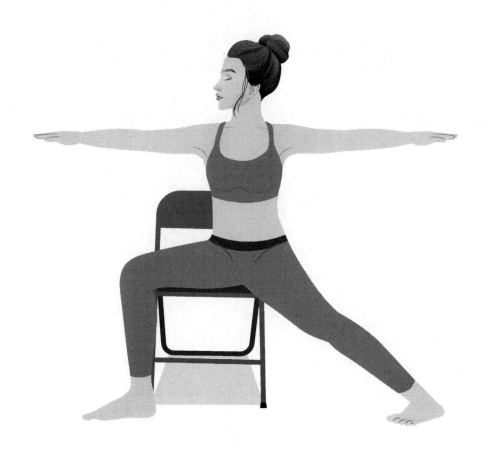

Instructions

1. Relax and recover from previous poses by sitting comfortably.

2. Keep your posture straight and move toward the left end of the chair.

3. Now, take your right leg out toward the right side of the chair and keep it at a 90-degree angle.

4. Move the left leg toward the left side of the chair and lengthen it to stretch it straight.

5. Raise your arms, so they reach a parallel position to the ground.

6. Move them upward, so that your fingers point to the ceiling.

7. Hold this position for 3-4 deep breaths and slowly come to the original relaxing pose.

8. Repeat the pose by starting with the left leg.

Benefits

- Strengthens legs, core, and ankles
- Improves balance
- Stretches hips, shoulders, and chest

Modification: After pointing fingers toward the ceiling, do not stop there; keep moving your arms toward your left side and stretch your belly muscles.

Safety Tip: Ensure you find a balance first, then proceed with the pose.

Seated Backbend Pose

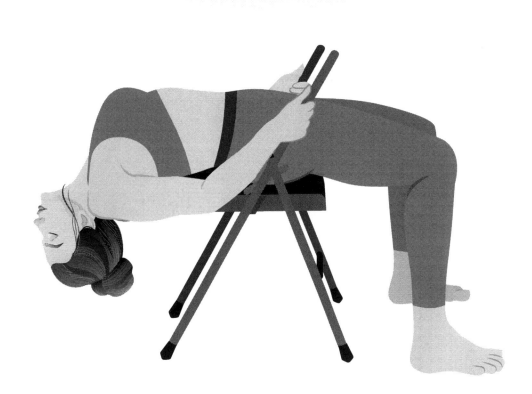

Instructions

1. This is an advanced-level pose that needs extra care. So, start when you're mentally and physically prepared.

2. Take a backless chair.

3. Sit in the chair to face its back with your legs on the side.

4. Now, raise one of your legs and pass it through the back of the chair.

5. Raise the other leg and do the same.

6. Keep your legs at a 90-degree angle.

7. Your chest is touching the back stand of the chair.

8. Now, slowly bend backward so your head is parallel to your legs.

9. At this stage, your chest is fully stretched, and your back covers the sitting area of the chair.

10. Hold this position for 3-4 deep breaths or as long as you feel comfortable.

11. Now, slowly move back to the original positions, starting with raising your head.

Benefits

- It opens up the chest and shoulders
- Improves spine flexibility
- Strengthens core muscles
- Improves digestive system

Modification: You can stretch your legs and take the support of the wall.

Safety Measure: Ensure you do not have a neck or head injury.

Side Stretch with Bended Arms

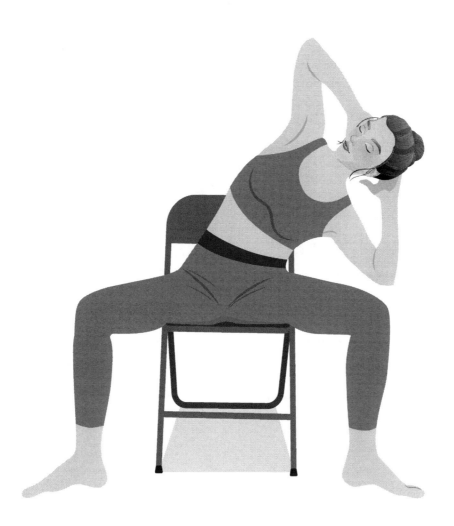

Instructions

1. Sit in the chair with your back stretched and place your hands on your knees.

2. Now, slowly move your legs to the sides of the chair so that your thighs become parallel to the ground.

3. Raise your arms and hold them parallel to the ground, then bend

them and place them behind your head.

4. Inhale and move your upper body toward the left side of the chair. This will give the right side of your body a perfect stretch.

5. Exhale and move your upper body back to the center of your body.

6. Inhale and repeat this movement toward the right side of your body.

7. Exhale and move it back to the center of your body.

8. Repeat this movement for 4-5 breaths.

Benefits

- Lengthens the spine and side muscles
- Improves flexibility in the torso and shoulders
- Stimulates the organs

Modification: Instead of moving sideways, move your body down to the ground.

Safety Measure: Ensure that there is not any arch or curl in your spine.

Chair Pigeon Pose

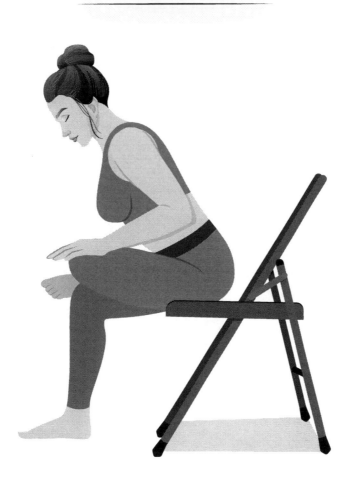

Instructions

1. Sit in a relaxing position in the chair.

2. Keep your legs at a 90-degree angle and keep your feet firm on the ground.

3. Raise your left leg and place your left ankle on the right thigh.

4. Inhale, then lean forward and keep your spine straight.

5. Exhale and put pressure on your left leg with your hands.

6. Repeat this position for 4-5 deep breaths.

7. Now, do this pose by starting with the other leg.

Benefits

- Stretches the glutes, hips, and thighs
- Improves hip mobility
- Increases circulation in the legs

Modification: You can lean forward such that your chest touches your leg.

Safety Tip: Keep your back straight throughout this pose.

Chair Locust Pose

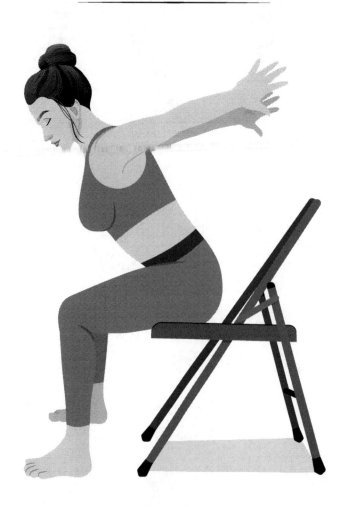

Instructions

1. Sit in a relaxing position in the chair.
2. Keep your legs at a 90-degree angle and keep your feet firm on the ground.
3. Inhale, then lean forward and keep your spine straight.
4. Stretch your arm backward and open your fingers.
5. Take deep breaths and hold this pose for 4-5 breaths.

Benefits

- Strengthens back muscles
- Stretches the chest and shoulders
- Improves core stability
- Improves the digestive system

Modification: You can lean forward down in a way that your chest touches your thighs and your fingers point to the ceiling.

Safety Measure: Ensure your shoulders are straight and your back is stretched.

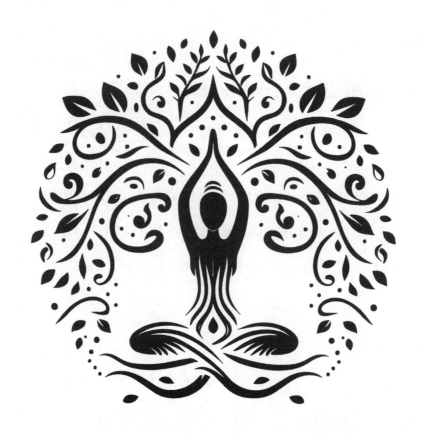

CHAPTER 6

A Holistic Approach to Weight Loss

This chapter covers how nutrition, mindful eating, and stress reduction can be combined with your chair yoga exercises to offer a holistic weight-loss approach. It also points out why paying attention to your body's natural hunger and fullness signals is essential to help develop healthier eating habits.

Nutrition for Weight Loss

Weight loss occurs with a calorie-deficit diet—meaning that the number of calories burned is greater than the calories consumed. Furthermore, our calorie consumption levels and satisfaction levels after eating are linked to what we eat. Scientifically backed dietary habits that may help you with weight loss include the following:

- Whole foods are lower in calories and even more filling than processed meals. One study discovered that people who ate more whole meals lost an additional 0.5 kg more weight per week than people who ate more processed meals.
- Fiber helps you eat fewer calories during the day. According to a study, people who took a high dietary fiber eating pattern for a six-month eating plan, lost 4.3 kg and 9.5 lbs. more weight than those who took low dietary fiber eating patterns programs.
- Protein helps you increase your muscle mass and burn more calories while resting.
- Fat in oil, avocado, and nut products can help you feel full and stop unwanted food cravings.
- Research has shown that people who drink 500ml of water before meals consume fewer calories than those who do not consume water.
- Consider these facts and remember that your nutrition is as essential for weight loss as chair yoga.

28-Day Meal Plan

The following meal plan has been developed for demonstrative purposes within a general calorie range suitable for weight management. It is not a replacement for specialized and individualized professional advice, as caloric requirements change depending on age, level of physical activity, gender, and desired weight loss.

'Week 1'

Breakfast	Snack 1	Lunch	Snack 2	Dinner
Day 1				
300-400 cal. Oatmeal with berries, nuts, and a teaspoon of honey	100-200 cal. Greek yogurt with a banana, sprinkled with chia seeds	400-500 cal. Grilled chicken breast sandwich on whole-wheat bread with lettuce, tomato, and avocado. A side of salad, vinaigrette dressing	100-200 cal. Walnuts, almonds, cranberries	500-600 cal. Salmon with lemon and herbs, vegetables roasted in the oven (broccoli, carrots), brown rice
Day 2				
300-400 cal. Oatmeal with berries, nuts, and a teaspoon of honey	100-200 cal. Greek yogurt with a banana, sprinkled with chia seeds	400-500 cal. Grilled chicken breast sandwich on whole-wheat bread with lettuce, tomato, and avocado. A side of salad, vinaigrette dressing	100-200 cal. Walnuts, almonds, cranberries	500-600 cal. Salmon with lemon and herbs, vegetables roasted in the oven (broccoli, carrots), brown rice
Day 3				
300-400 cal. Scrambled eggs, spinach, whole wheat roll	100-200 cal. Coffee with a sprinkling of cinnamon spice	400-500 cal. Lentil soup with a whole wheat roll, simple salad	100-200 cal. Carrot, broccoli, cauliflower bunches	500-600 cal. Turkey chili with low-fat Greek yogurt, avocado toppings
Day 4				
300-400 cal. Oatmeal with berries, nuts, and a teaspoon of honey	100-200 cal. Greek yogurt with a banana, sprinkled with chia seeds	400-500 cal. Grilled chicken breast sandwich on whole-wheat bread with lettuce, tomato, and avocado. A side of salad, vinaigrette dressing	100-200 cal. Walnuts, almonds, cranberries	500-600 cal. Salmon with lemon and herbs, vegetables roasted in the oven (broccoli, carrots), brown rice
Day 5				
300-400 cal. Oatmeal with berries, nuts, and a teaspoon of honey	100-200 cal. Greek yogurt with a banana, sprinkled with chia seeds	400-500 cal. Grilled chicken breast sandwich on whole-wheat bread with lettuce, tomato, and avocado. A side of salad, vinaigrette dressing	100-200 cal. Walnuts, almonds, cranberries	500-600 cal. Salmon with lemon and herbs, vegetables roasted in the oven (broccoli, carrots), brown rice
Day 6				
300-400 cal. Scrambled eggs, spinach, whole wheat roll	100-200 cal. Coffee with a sprinkling of cinnamon spice	400-500 cal. Lentil soup with a whole wheat roll, simple salad	100-200 cal. Carrot, broccoli, cauliflower bunches	500-600 cal. Turkey chili with low-fat Greek yogurt, avocado toppings
Day 7				
300-400 cal. Oatmeal with berries, nuts, and a teaspoon of honey	100-200 cal. Greek yogurt with a banana, sprinkled with chia seeds	400-500 cal. Grilled chicken breast sandwich on whole-wheat bread with lettuce, tomato, and avocado. A side of salad, vinaigrette dressing	100-200 cal. Walnuts, almonds, cranberries	500-600 cal. Salmon with lemon and herbs, vegetables roasted in the oven (broccoli, carrots), brown rice

'Week 2'

Breakfast	Snack 1	Lunch	Snack 2	Dinner
		Day 1		
		Day 2		
		Day 3		
		Day 4		
		Day 5		
		Day 6		
		Day 7		

'Week 3'

Breakfast	Snack 1	Lunch	Snack 2	Dinner
		Day 1		
		Day 2		
		Day 3		
		Day 4		
		Day 5		
		Day 6		
		Day 7		

'Week 4'

Breakfast	Snack 1	Lunch	Snack 2	Dinner
		Day 1		
		Day 2		
		Day 3		
		Day 4		
		Day 5		
		Day 6		
		Day 7		

Weeks 2, 3, and 4

Maintain the structure as indicated while experimenting with variations to make your meal plan more exciting. Customize your plan and eat batches of breakfast and lunch as follows:

- Switch to whole-wheat pancakes with berries and low-fat yogurt. You may also have whole-wheat waffles served with nut butter and banana slices.
- Try a whole-wheat bun with a black bean burger patty, lettuce, tomato, and avocado. Alternatively, you may serve lentil pasta salad with chopped vegetables and light vinaigrette as an accompaniment.
- Choose sliced bell peppers with hummus, a small pear, and a slice of string cheese.
- Consume a sheet of tofu baked with roasted Brussels sprouts, quinoa, or grilled shrimp with whole-wheat couscous and steamed asparagus.
- Cook your food at home for more controlled ingredients and portions.

Substituting these options based on nutrient content allows you to personalize your meal plan. Meal portions should stick to the recommended levels noted above. Always have plenty of water throughout the day.

Mindful Eating

Mindful eating is about developing a Zen consciousness of the moment by consuming food. You can use it as a tool to distinguish between real hunger and thinking about your emotions around food. It should build a more stable emotional attitude toward food. Here's how you can start:

- Create a relaxing environment. Turn off the television or phone, eat meals at a table, and pay attention to when and what you consume.

- Feel with your senses. Look at your food and note the colors, textures, smells, and flavors. Chew slowly and enjoy each bite.

- Note when you are comfortable eating. Ask yourself, "Am I hungry, or am I bored, worried, or stressed?" Only eat once you're hungry.

- Act without judgment. There are no such items as "good" and "bad" foods.

- Express gratefulness. Before you begin eating, think about what went into making that dish: the rain that fed the crop, the sunshine that warmed it, and the time it took to locate, obtain, clean, and prepare it. Consider the time and effort that went into meal planning.

Be mindful of every bite you take.

Stress Management for Weight Loss

Regular levels of constant stress can harm any weight loss program. The better way to eliminate your stress levels and support your struggle with unwanted extra pounds includes:

- **Identifying your sources of stress:** To understand what triggers stress the most, start with something simple like journaling to find any patterns.

- **Learning and regularly practicing mindfulness methods:** Use meditation, progressive muscle relaxation, or deep breathing techniques to experience mind and body healing as often as possible.

- **Exercising daily:** Use physical activity as a natural anti-stress method. You can choose from various fun activities, such as walking, dancing, yoga, and more.

- **Developing healthy sleep habits:** Try to go to bed and wake up at the same time every day to get 7-8 hours of sleep every night. Develop a quiet and pleasantly relaxing evening routine, after which falling asleep will be very easy.

- **Seeking social support:** Find support from the family, join a local support group or seek therapy.

Listening to Your Body

Our bodies talk to us all the time. Understanding your body's hunger and fullness clues is essential for weight management. Here is how you can listen to your body's inner voice:

- Accurate hunger signals take a long time to become apparent. Cravings, conversely, seem to appear out of nowhere, inspired by emotions or routine.

- Body Examination is a procedure that involves observation. Before eating, take time to examine your body. Are there any bodily sensations of hunger when your stomach growls or your energy decreases?

- Avoid excessive emotions, like stress, frustration, or tedium, prompting you to eat negligently.

- It takes a few minutes for your stomach to apprise your brain of how stuffed you are, so eat with attention and end before having no more room in your belly.

- Avoid depriving yourself of food; eat moderately and maintain a healthy diet.

Remember, mindfulness, tension control, and listening to your body are intertwined—they collaborate to make practical and beneficial weight loss and living practical goals.

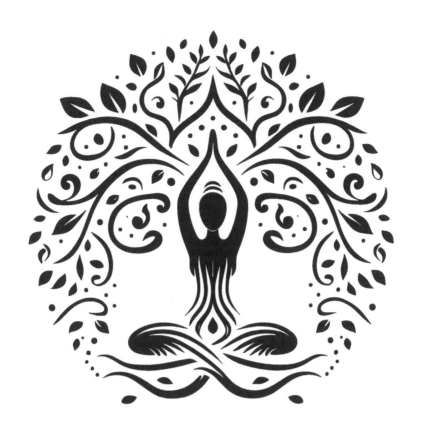

CHAPTER 7

Your 28-Day
Chair Yoga Routine

The 28-day plan in this chapter includes poses from all exercises related to belly fat, mobility, and flexibility to provide a well-rounded routine. Listen to your body and adjust repetitions or rest as needed.

'Your 28-Day Chair Yoga Routine'

	Day 1 Belly Fat Focus	Day 2 Mobility Focus	Day 3 Belly Fat Focus	Day 4 Mobility Focus	Day 5 Flexibility Focus	Day 6	Day 7 Challenge yourself with advanced belly fat poses
Week 1 Focus (4 Minutes)	Seated Side Stretch–3 repetitions on each side (hold for 5 breaths) Cat-Cow Stretch–5 repetitions Forward Bend–3 repetitions (hold for 5 breaths) Seated Spinal Twists–3 repetitions on each side (hold for 5 breaths)	Seated Neck Stretch–3 repetitions on each side (hold for 5 breaths) Seated Hip Circles–5 repetitions in each direction Chair March–3 repetitions on each leg Cross Body Punch–5 repetitions on each side	Seated Side Stretch–3 repetitions on each side (hold for 5 breaths) Cat-Cow Stretch–5 repetitions Forward Bend–3 repetitions (hold for 5 breaths) Seated Spinal Twists–3 repetitions on each side (hold for 5 breaths)	Seated Neck Stretch–3 repetitions on each side (hold for 5 breaths) Seated Hip Circles–5 repetitions in each direction Chair March–3 repetitions on each leg Cross Body Punch–5 repetitions on each side	Seated Hamstring Stretch–3 repetitions on each side (hold for 5 breaths) Seated Hero's Pose - Hold for as long as comfortable (30 seconds to 1 minute) Seated Inner Thigh Stretch–3 repetitions on each side (hold for 5 breaths)	Rest	Chair Boat Pose–3 repetitions Chair Plank–3 repetitions Chair Reverse Warrior–3 repetitions Seated Bicycle Crunches–3 repetitions
	Day 8 Belly Fat Focus	Day 9 Mobility Focus	Day 10 Belly Fat Focus	Day 11 Mobility Focus	Day 12 Flexibility Focus	Day 13	Day 14 Challenge yourself with advanced belly fat poses
Week 2	Seated Side Stretch–3 repetitions on each side (hold for 5 breaths) Cat-Cow Stretch–5 repetitions Forward Bend–3 repetitions (hold for 5 breaths) Seated Spinal Twists–3 repetitions on each side (hold for 5 breaths)	Seated Neck Stretch–3 repetitions on each side (hold for 5 breaths) Seated Hip Circles–5 repetitions in each direction Chair March–3 repetitions on each leg Cross Body Punch–5 repetitions on each side Reach out to Your Thigh–3 repetitions	Seated Side Stretch–3 repetitions on each side (hold for 5 breaths) Cat-Cow Stretch–5 repetitions Forward Bend–3 repetitions (hold for 5 breaths) Seated Spinal Twists–3 repetitions on each side (hold for 5 breaths)	Seated Neck Stretch–3 repetitions on each side (hold for 5 breaths) Seated Hip Circles–5 repetitions in each direction Chair March–3 repetitions on each leg Cross Body Punch–5 repetitions on each side	Seated Hamstring Stretch–3 repetitions on each side (hold for 5 breaths) Seated Hero's Pose - Hold for as long as comfortable (30 seconds to 1 minute) Seated Inner Thigh Stretch–3 repetitions on each side (hold for 5 breaths) Chair Bicep Dips–3 repetitions	Rest	Chair Boat Pose–3 repetitions Chair Plank–3 repetitions Chair Reverse Warrior–3 repetitions Seated Bicycle Crunches–3 repetitions

Week 3	Day 15	Day 16	Day 17	Day 18	Day 19	Day 20	Day 21
	Belly Fat Focus	Mobility Focus	Belly Fat Focus	Mobility Focus	Flexibility Focus		Challenge yourself with advanced belly fat poses
	Seated Side Stretch–3 repetitions on each side (hold for 5 breaths) Cat-Cow Stretch–5 repetitions Forward Bend–3 repetitions (hold for 5 breaths) Seated Spinal Twists–3 repetitions on each side (hold for 5 breaths)	Seated Neck Stretch–3 repetitions on each side (hold for 5 breaths) Seated Hip Circles–5 repetitions in each direction Chair March–3 repetitions on each leg Cross Body Punch–5 repetitions on each side Reach out to Your Thigh–3 repetitions	Seated Side Stretch–3 repetitions on each side (hold for 5 breaths) Cat-Cow Stretch–5 repetitions Forward Bend–3 repetitions (hold for 5 breaths) Seated Spinal Twists–3 repetitions on each side (hold for 5 breaths) Chair Mountain Pose–3 repetitions	Seated Neck Stretch–3 repetitions on each side (hold for 5 breaths) Seated Hip Circles–5 repetitions in each direction Chair March–3 repetitions on each leg Cross Body Punch–5 repetitions on each side	Seated Hamstring Stretch–3 repetitions on each side (hold for 5 breaths) Seated Hero's Pose - Hold for as long as comfortable (30 seconds to 1 minute) Seated Inner Thigh Stretch–3 repetitions on each side (hold for 5 breaths) Chair Bicep Dips–3 repetitions	Rest	Chair Boat Pose–3 repetitions Chair Plank–3 repetitions Chair Reverse Warrior–3 repetitions Seated Bicycle Crunches–3 repetitions

Week 4	Day 22	Day 23	Day 24	Day 25	Day 26	Day 27	Day 26
	Challenge yourself with intermediate belly fat poses	Challenge yourself with intermediate mobility poses	Challenge yourself with intermediate belly fat poses	Challenge yourself with intermediate mobility poses	Challenge yourself with intermediate flexibility poses		Challenge yourself with advanced-level flexibility poses
	Seated Leg Lifts–3 repetitions for each leg Chair Eagle Pose–3 repetitions on each side (hold for 5 breaths) Seated Cow Face–3 repetitions on each side (hold for 5 breaths)	Seated Neck Rolls–5 repetitions in each direction (hold for 5 breaths) Chair Squats–5 repetitions Chair March–4 repetitions on each leg Cross Body Punch–6 repetitions on each side	Seated Leg Lifts–3 repetitions for each leg Chair Eagle Pose–3 repetitions on each side (hold for 5 breaths) Seated Cow Face–3 repetitions on each side (hold for 5 breaths)	Seated Neck Rolls–5 repetitions in each direction (hold for 5 breaths) Chair Squats–5 repetitions Chair March–4 repetitions on each leg Cross Body Punch–6 repetitions on each side	Goddess Pose–Hold for as long as comfortable (30 seconds to 1 minute) per side Seated Ankle Circles–5 repetitions in each direction Seated Shoulder Twists–5 repetitions in each direction (hold for 5 breaths)	Rest	Chair Warrior II Pose–2 repetitions Seated Backbend Pose –2 repetitions Side Stretch with Bent Arms–2 repetitions Chair Pigeon Pose–2 repetitions Chair Locust Pose–2 repetitions

The structure of your daily chair yoga routine should include:

Warm-up (2 Minutes)

Follow this warm-up before any exercise routine.

- Seated Neck Rolls–5 repetitions in each direction
- Seated Shoulder Rolls–5 repetitions forward and backward

Focus exercises (4 minutes)

Cool-down (2 Minutes)

Follow this cool-down routine after the daily workout.

- Deep Breaths (Seated): Inhale for four counts, exhale for six counts, and repeat five times.

Progression

Feel free to swap exercises within the focus sections (Belly Fat, Mobility, Flexibility) to create variety. If 10-minute duration feels easy, consider extending the hold times or adding an extra repetition.

Chair Yoga Habit Tracker

Monitor your daily yoga routine through this tracker. This will help you see how these factors combine to make you the healthiest possible. Be honest while monitoring your habits.

Date: ....

Chair Yoga Session Done? Yes/No:

_____

How did you feel during/after yoga today?

_____

What did you eat today?

_____

How many glasses of water did you have?

_____

How were you feeling all day?

_____

Did you have difficulty falling asleep?

_____

Are there any positive or negative thoughts related to chair yoga today?

_____

Did you make any plans to customize your program?

_____

Final Thoughts

To conclude this book, let me tell you this straightforward truth: the chair is not where you stop. It is the beginning. Once you develop a habit, everything seems a part of your daily life. So please, take everything we learned here—strength, flexibility, and mindfulness—and do not stop. Try yoga on the mat, and take it outside—the choice is yours and yours alone. Have an incredible 28-day journey, and may you breathe deep, move for the better, and develop your life potential.

About the Author

Semine T. is a certified yoga instructor with a vision to make yoga available to everyone, regardless of strength, weight, or age. She leads chair yoga classes, which promote strength, flexibility, well-being, and other advantages without requiring extensive floor work. She is enthusiastic about assisting adults in losing weight and explains how people can do so via chair yoga.

Made in the USA
Middletown, DE
14 September 2024